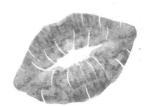

Dirty Talk
Phrases

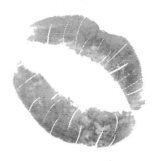

ADULT COLORING BOOK

THIS BOOK BELONGS TO:

_____

COLOR TEST PAGE

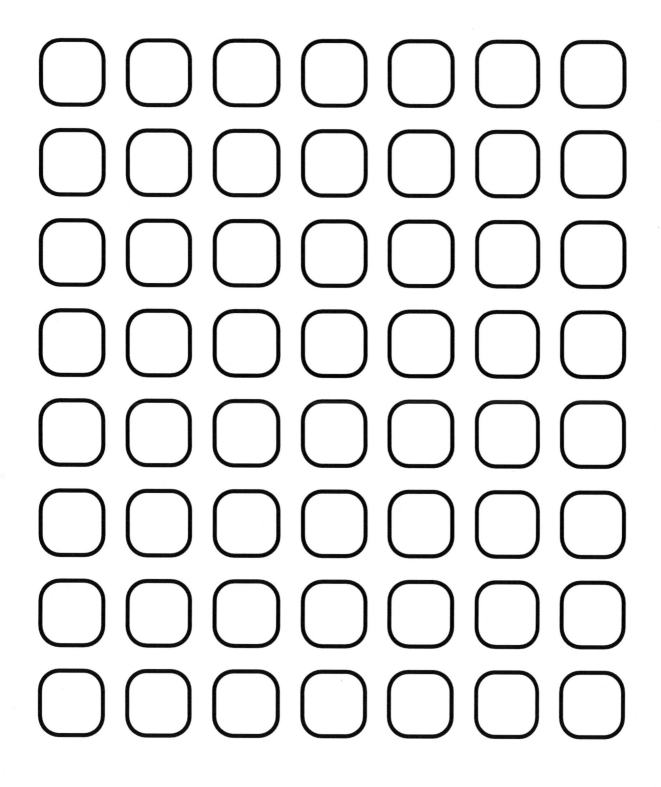

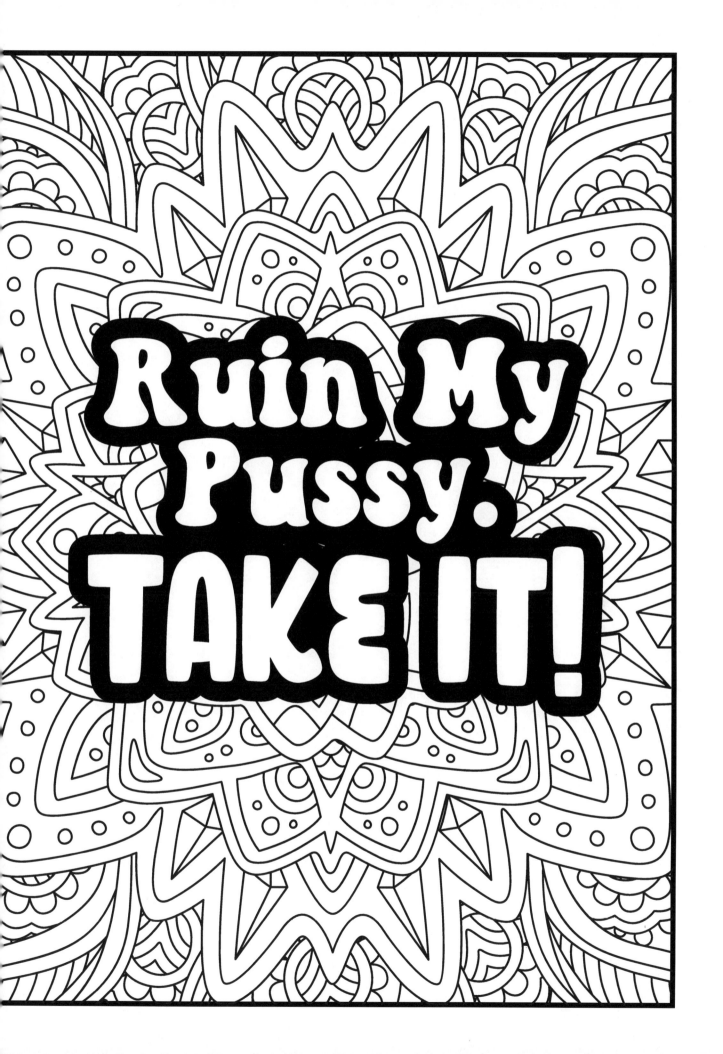

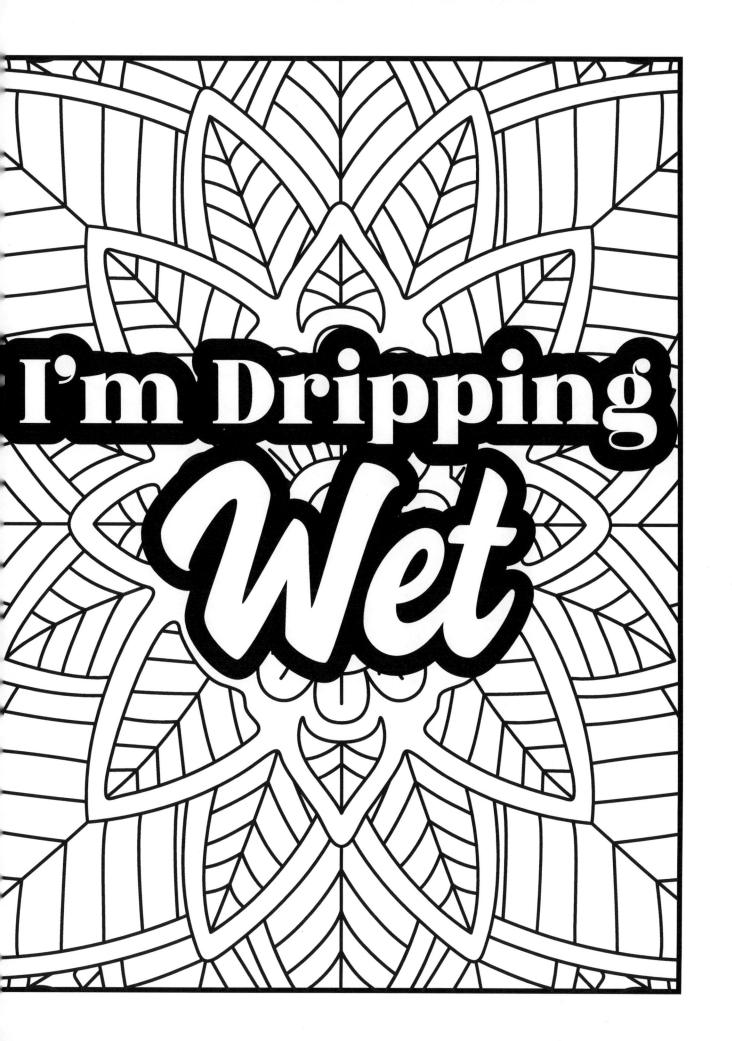

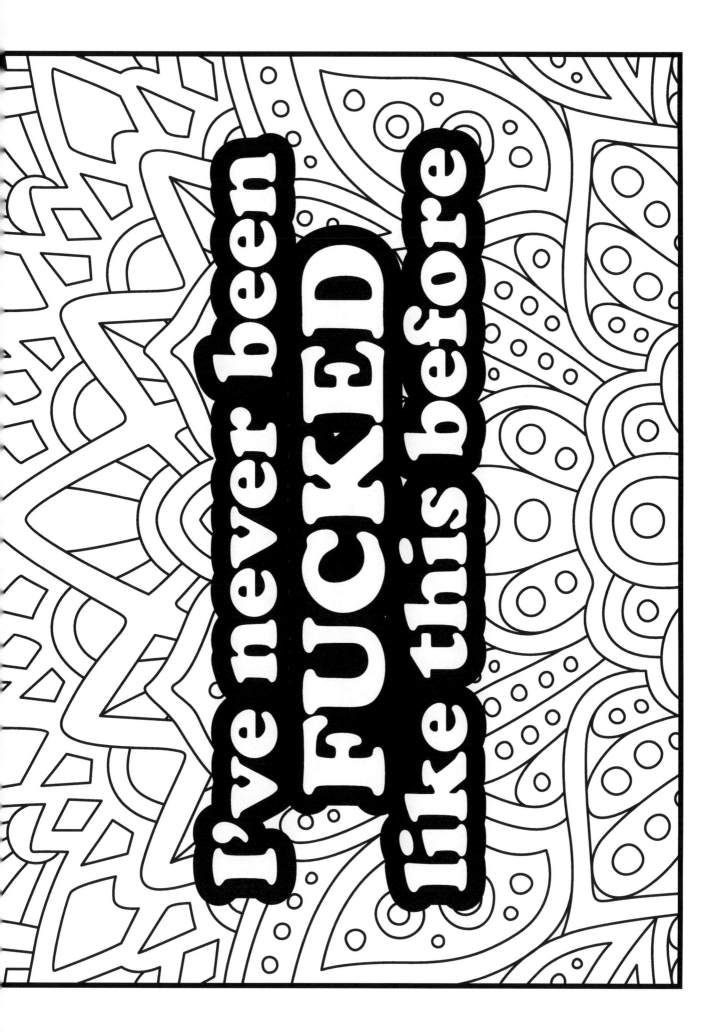

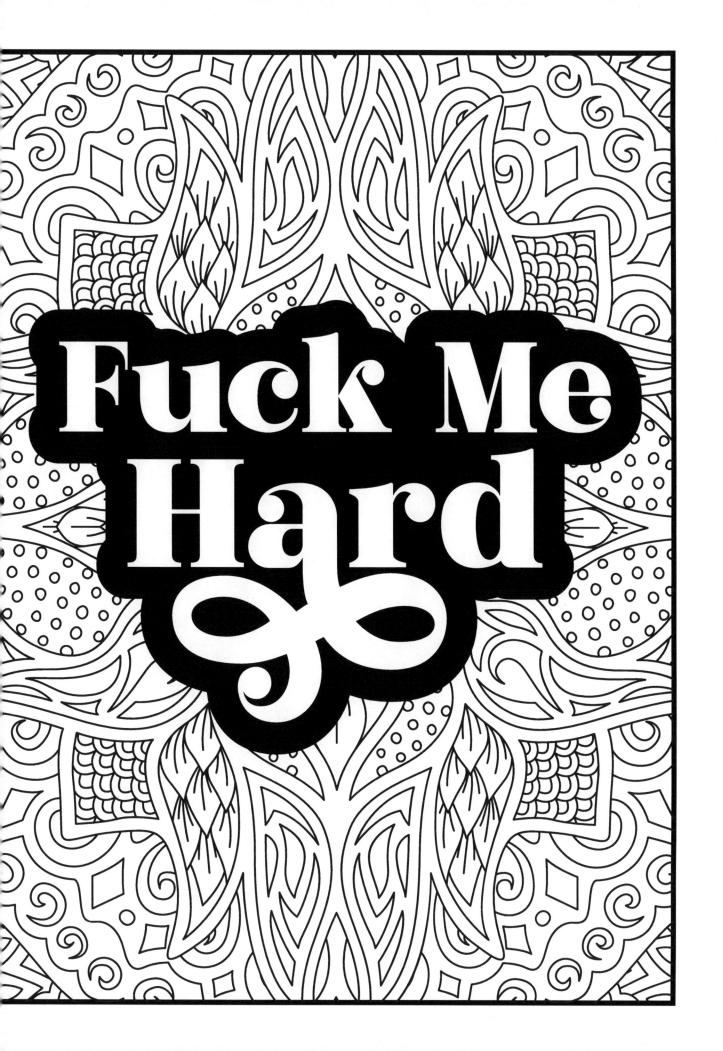

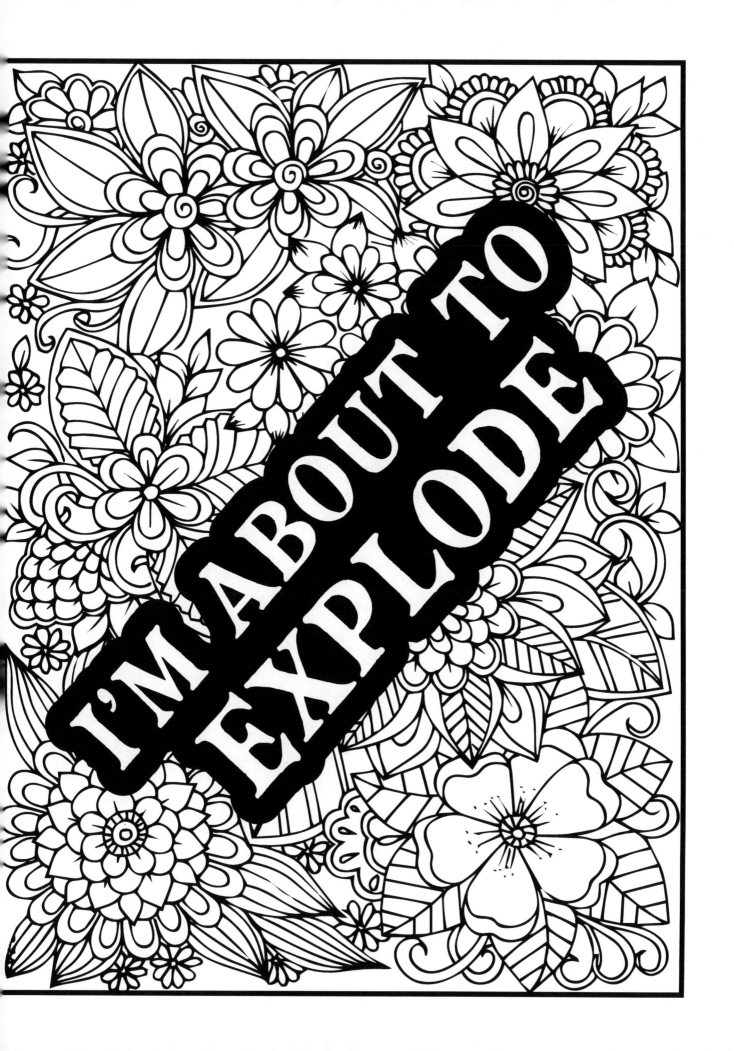

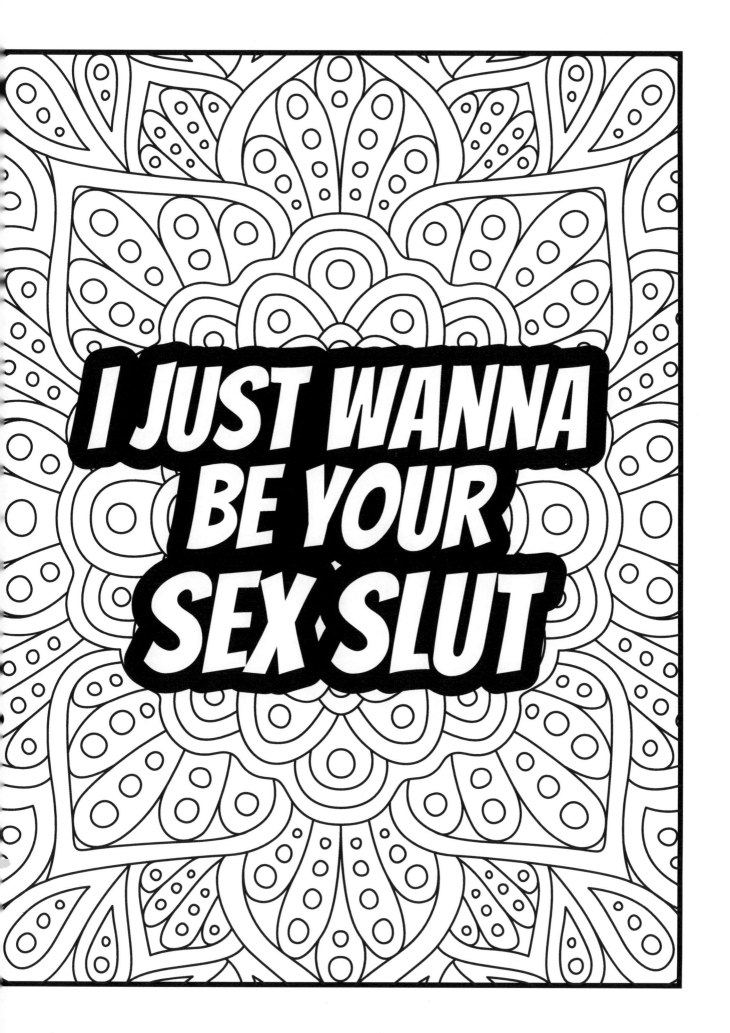

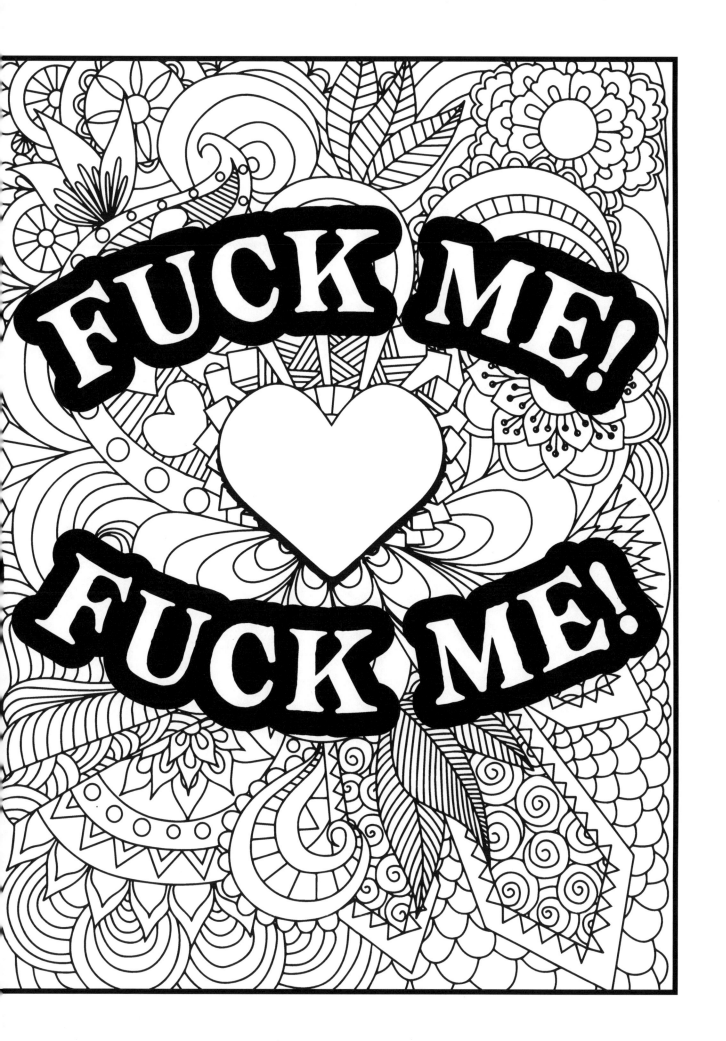

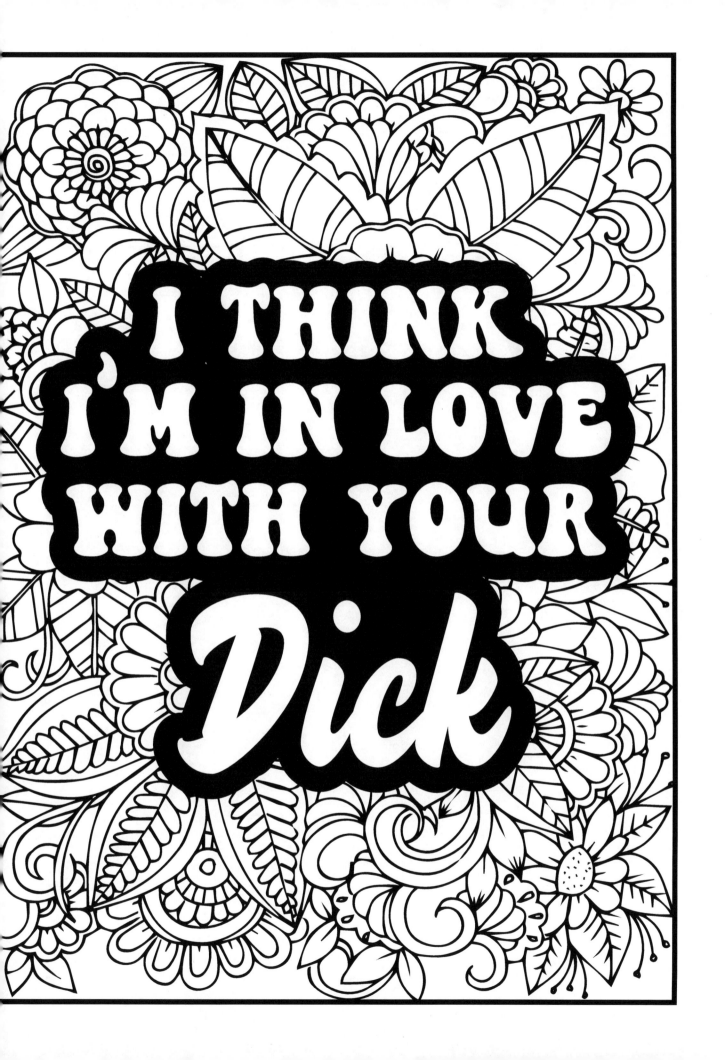

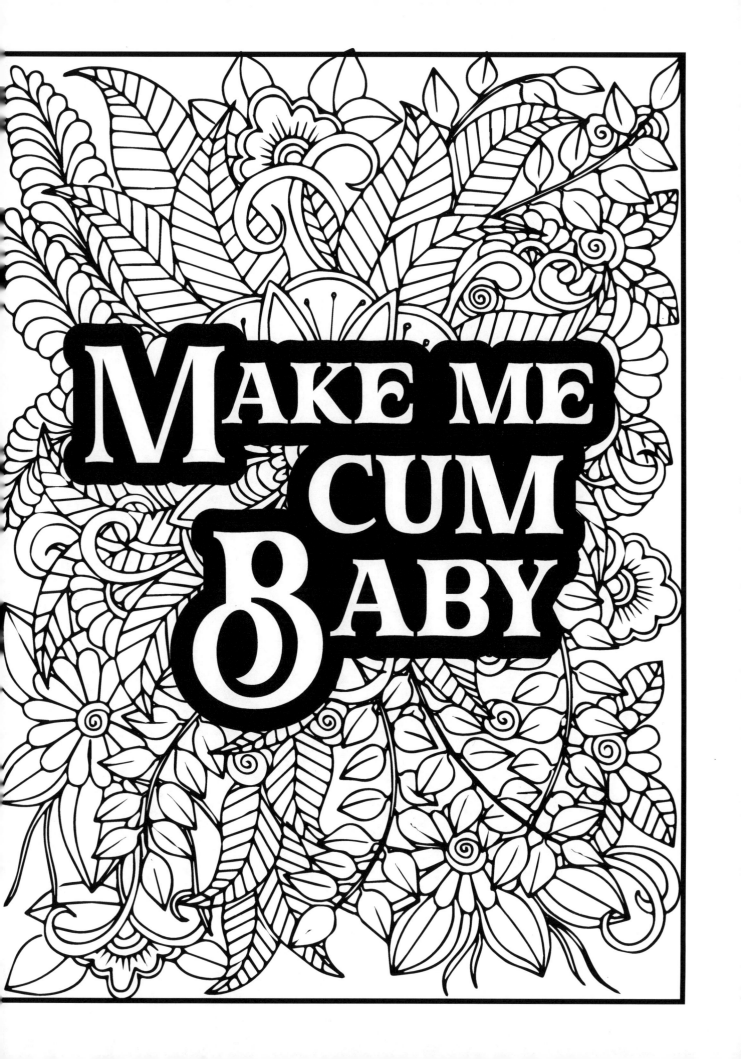

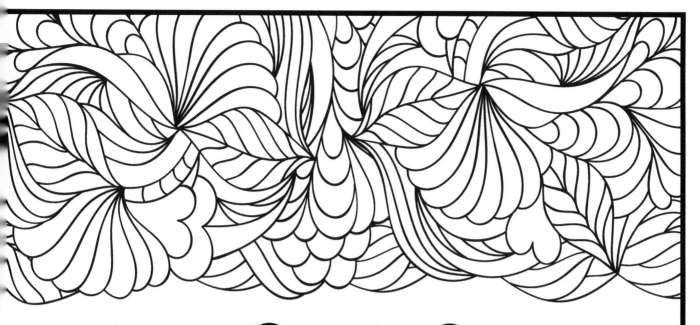

I'M GOING TO JERK YOU OFF UNTIL I GET EVERY LAST DROP OUT OF YOU

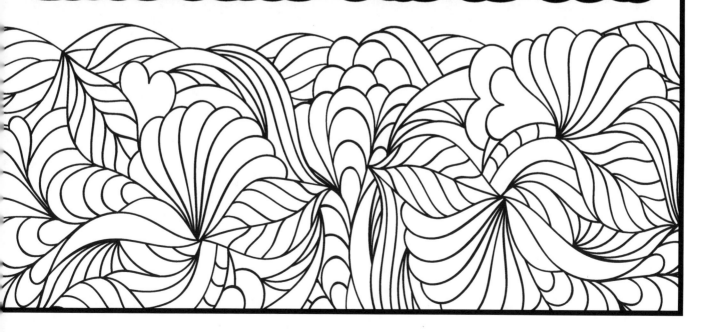

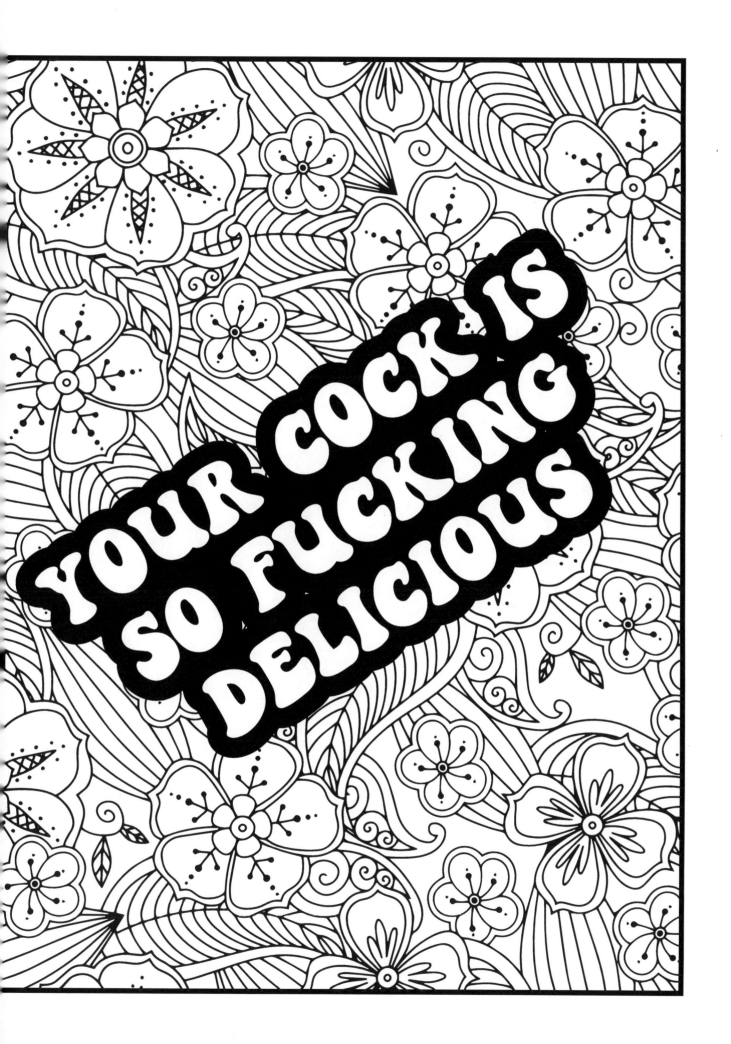

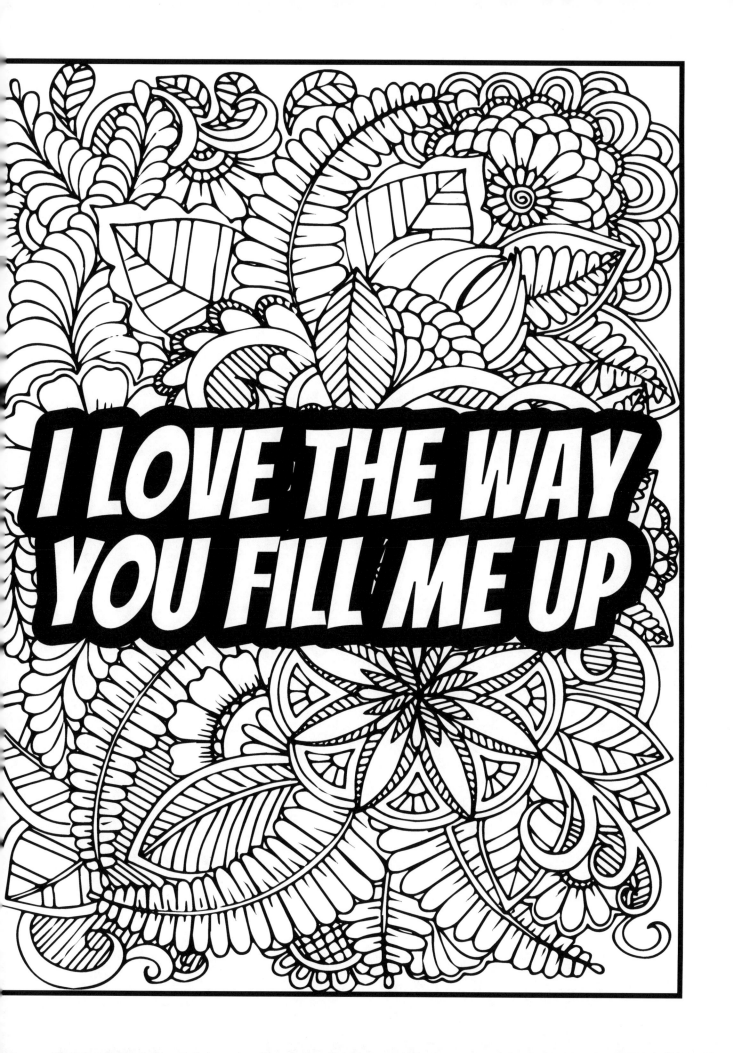

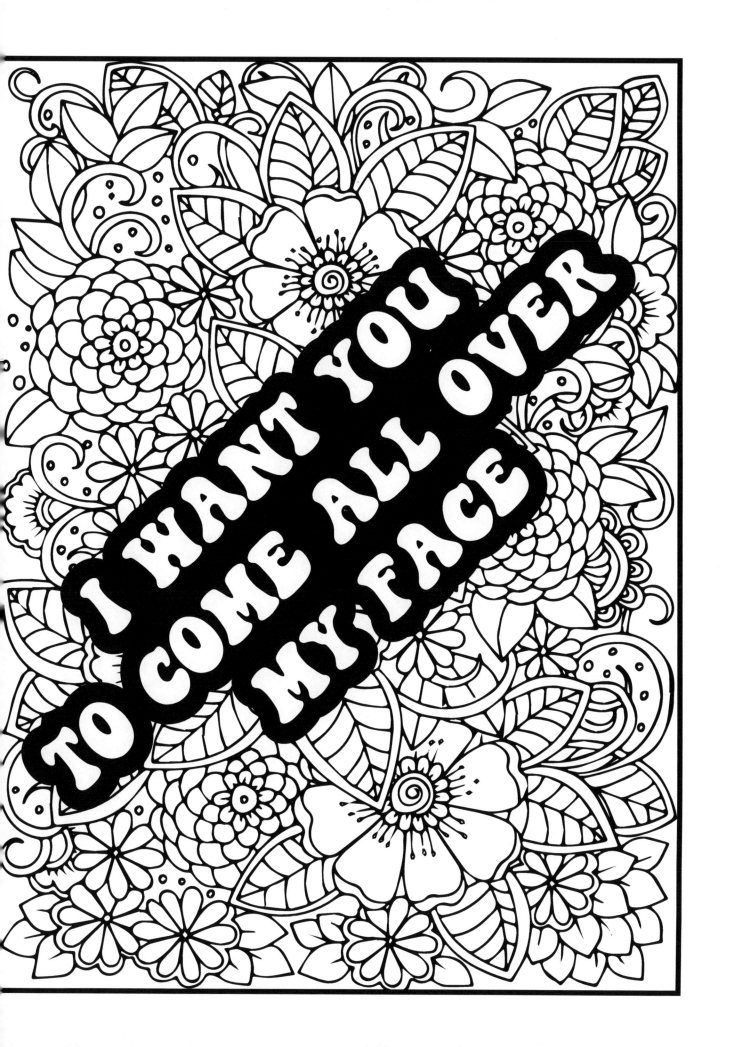

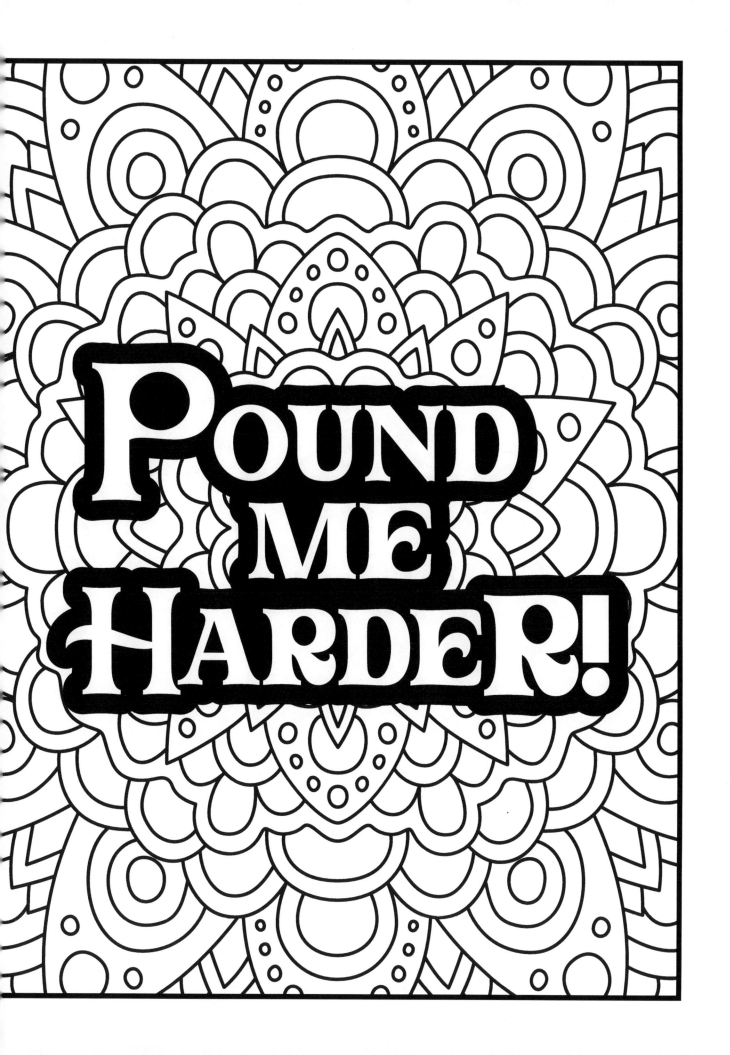

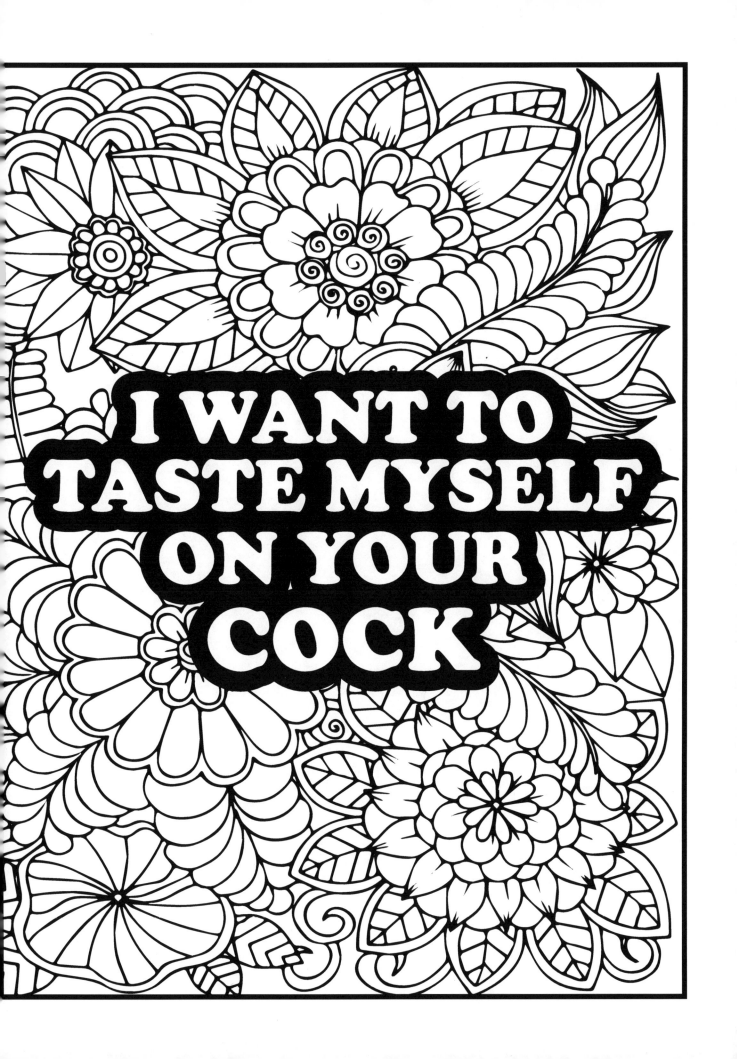

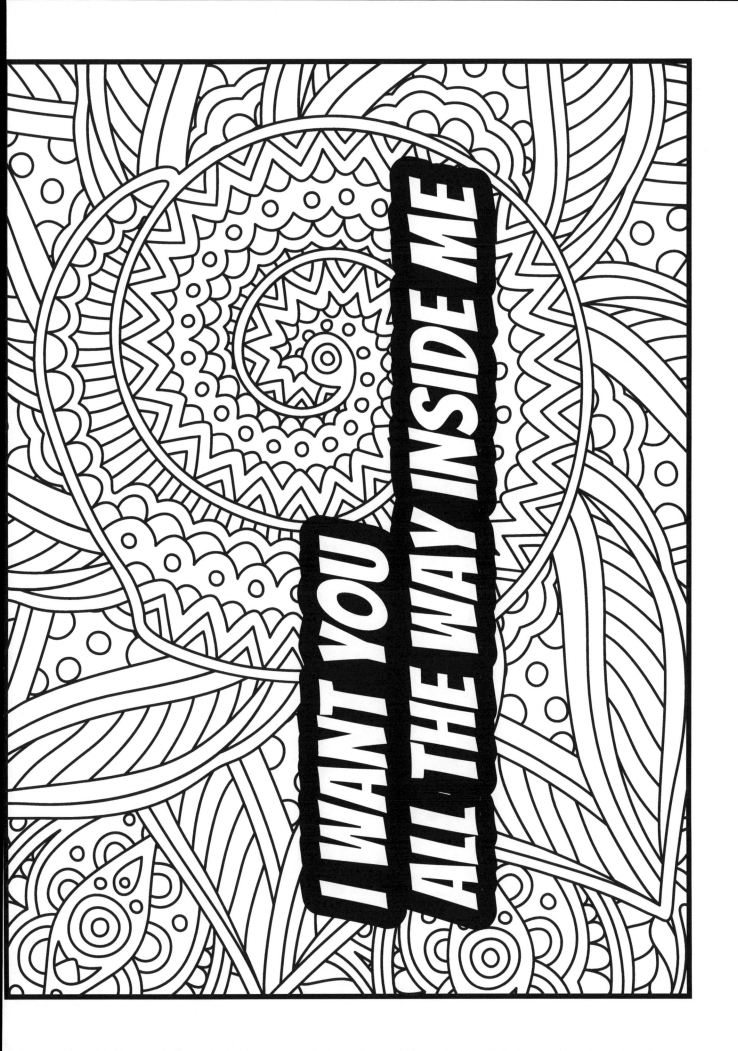

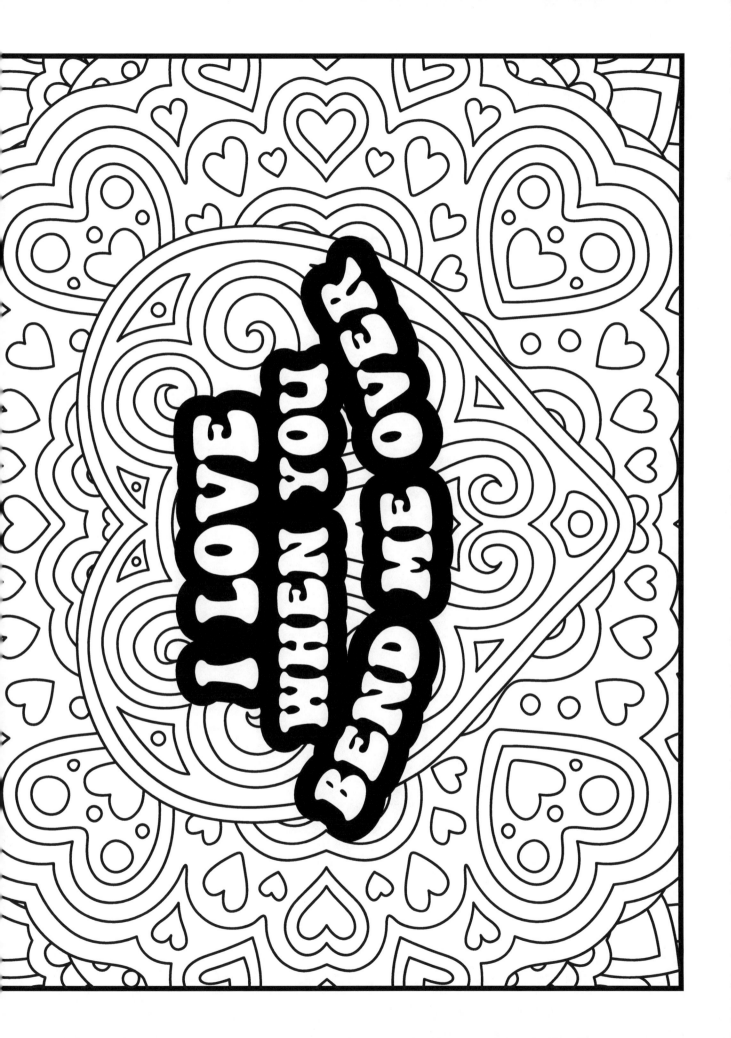

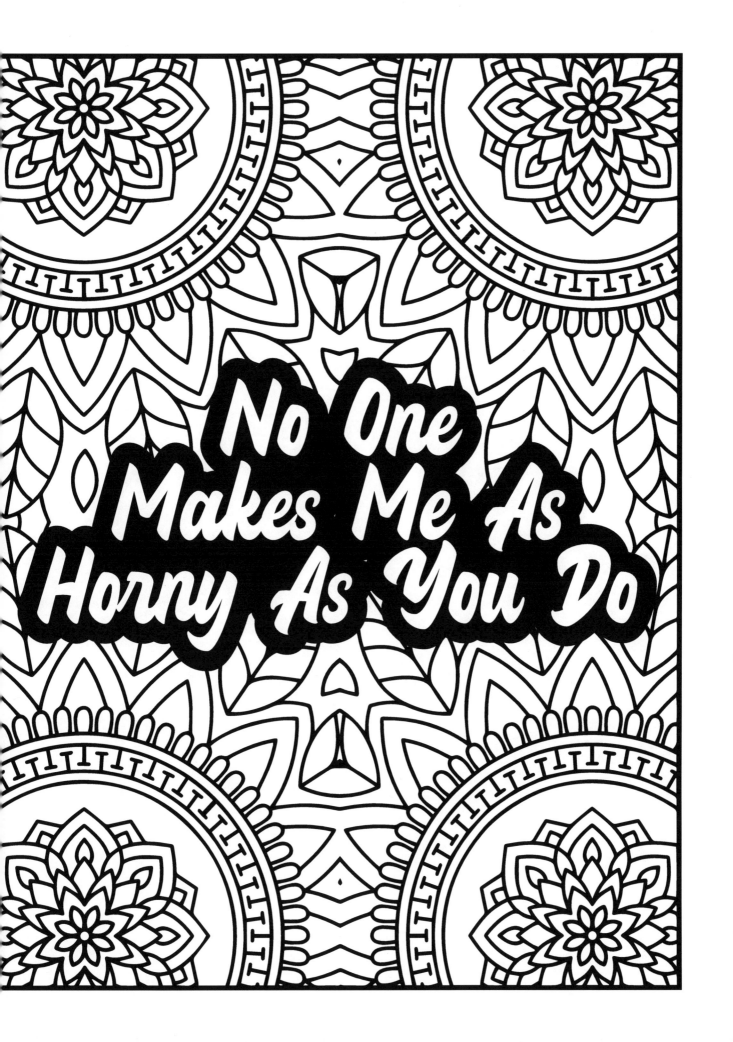

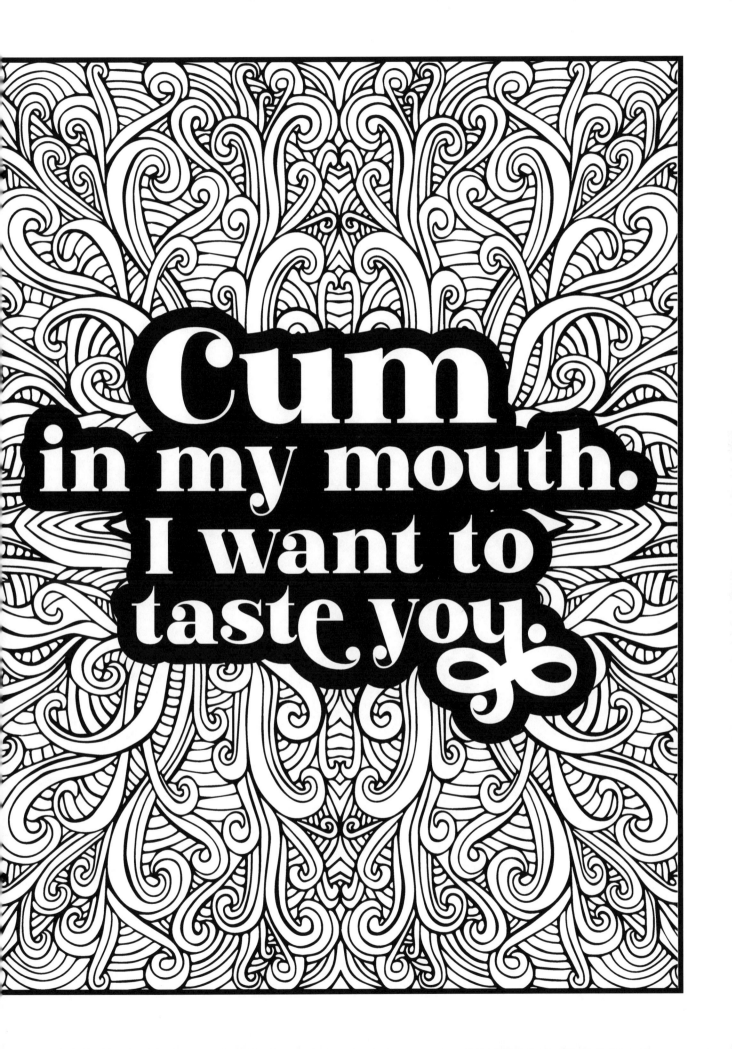

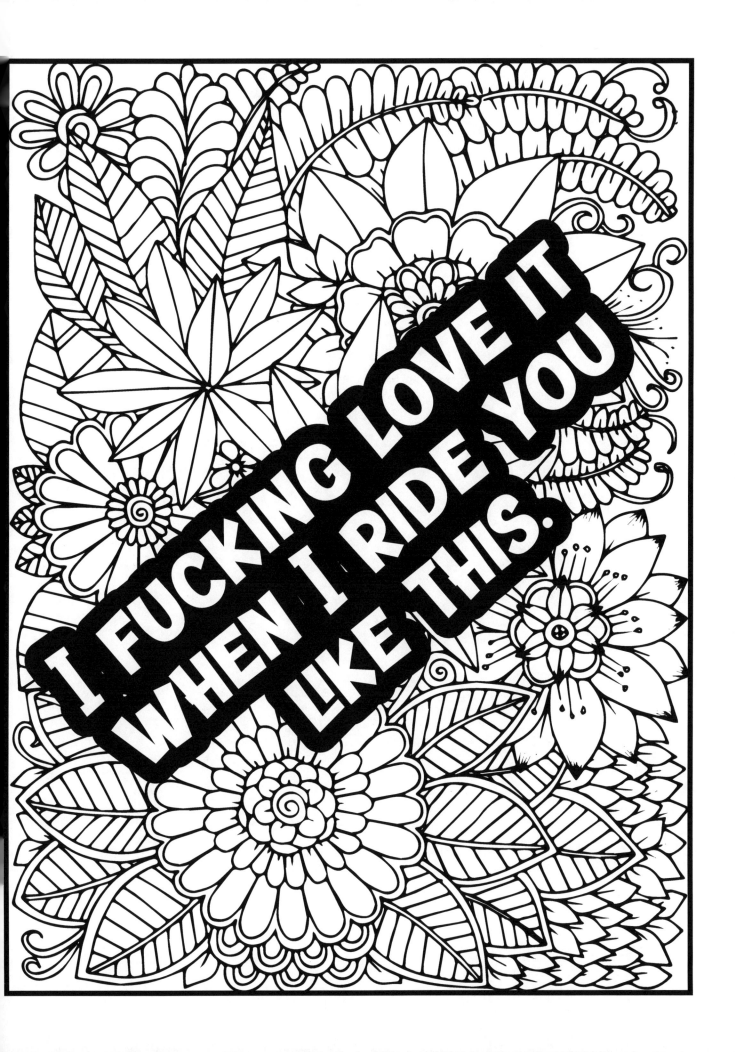

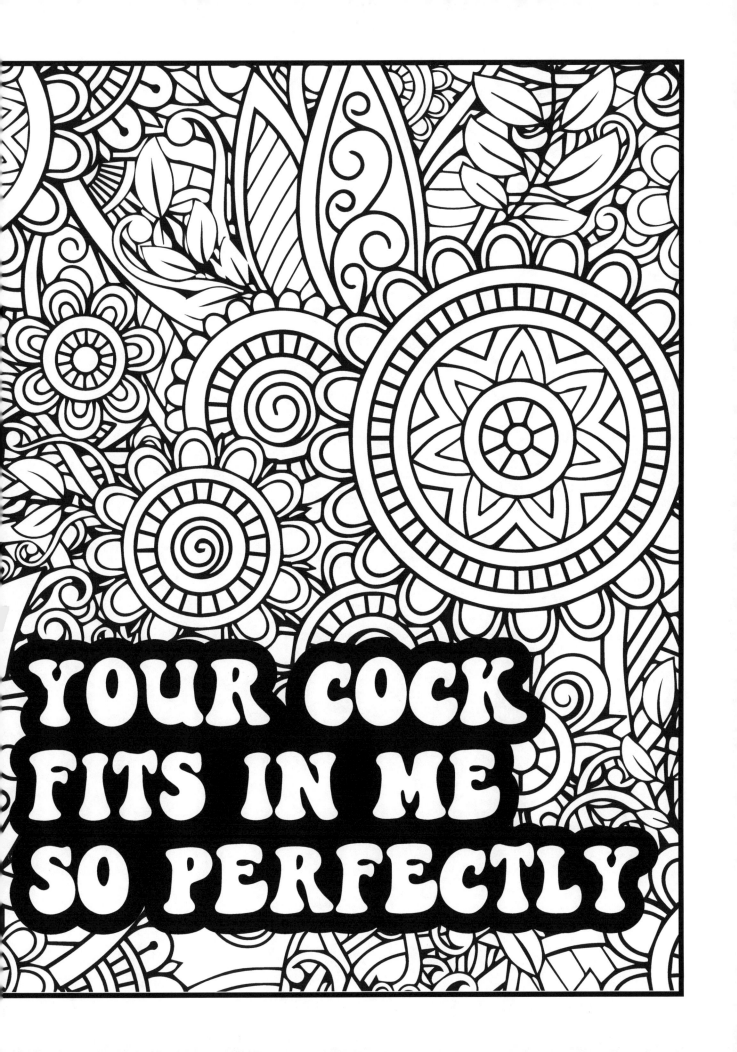

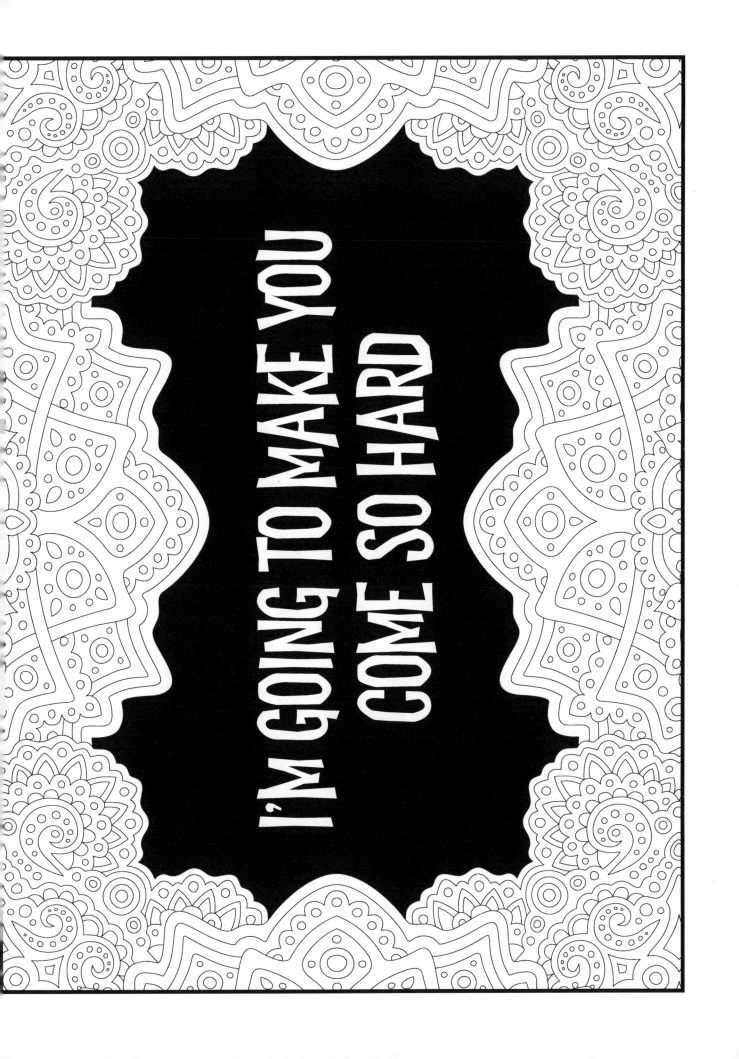

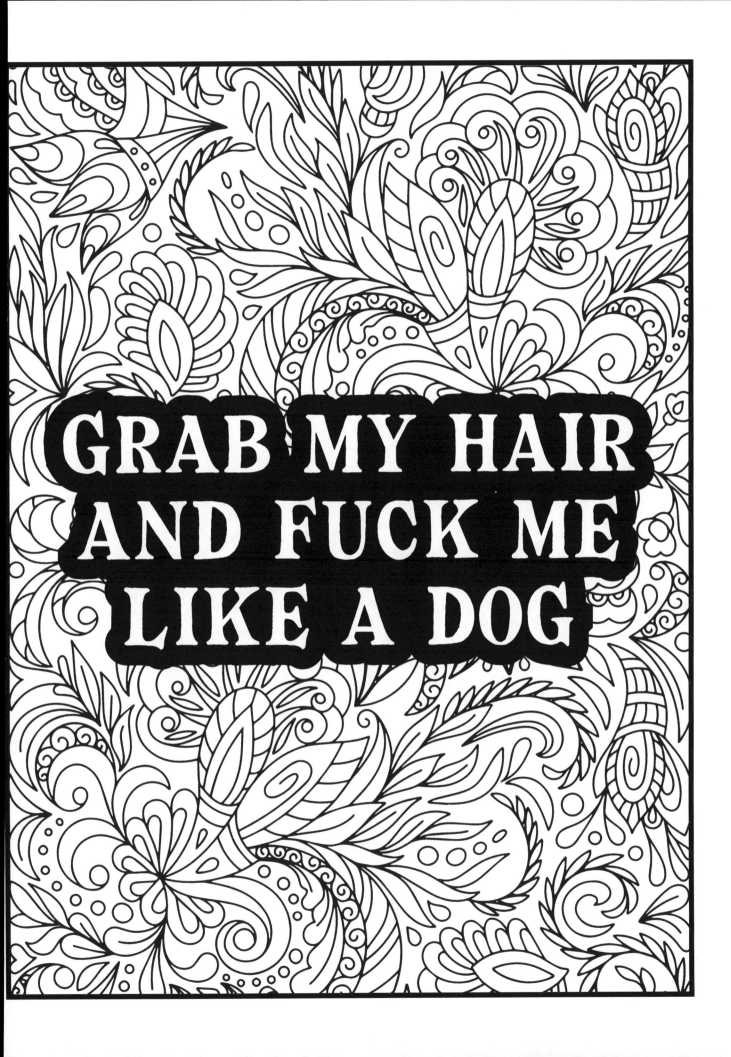

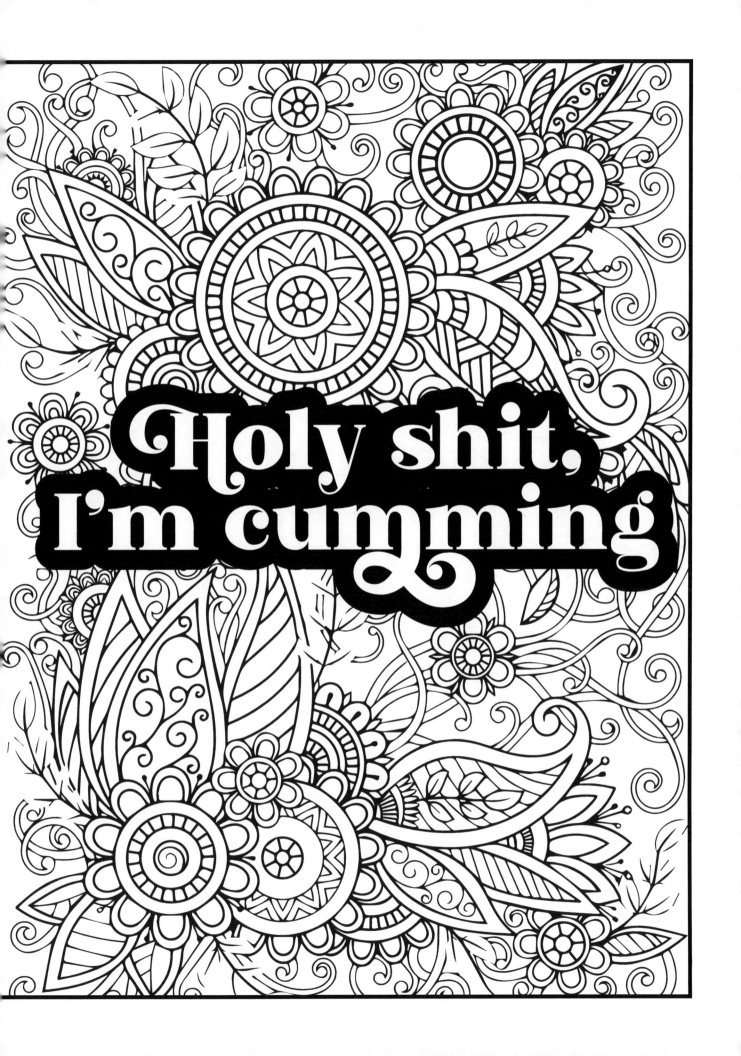

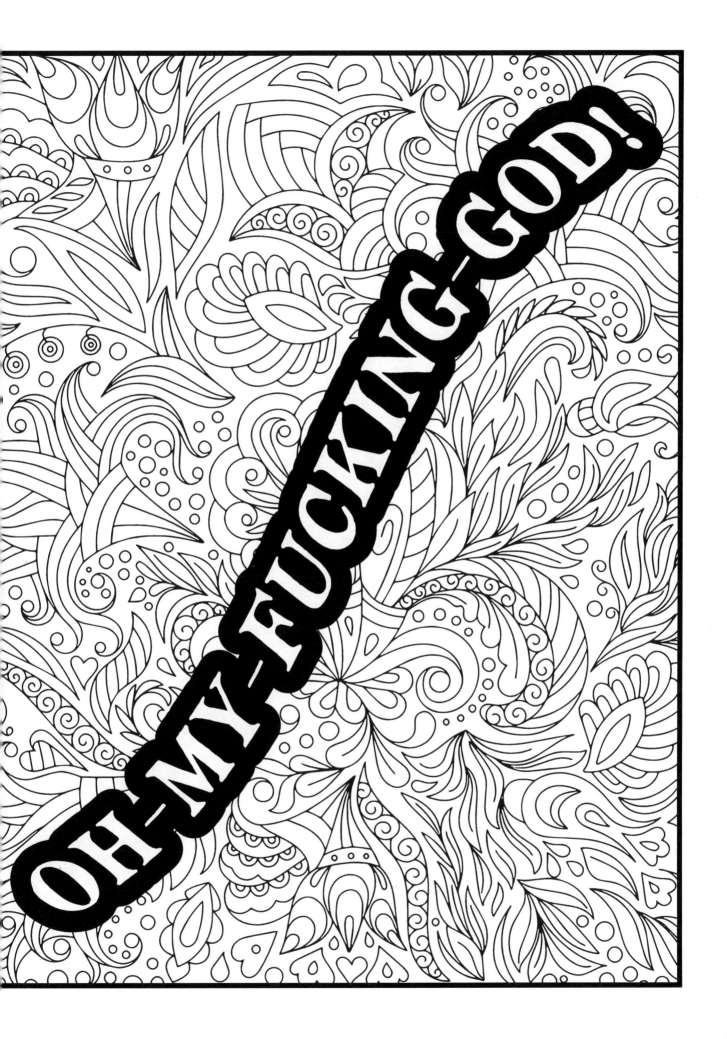

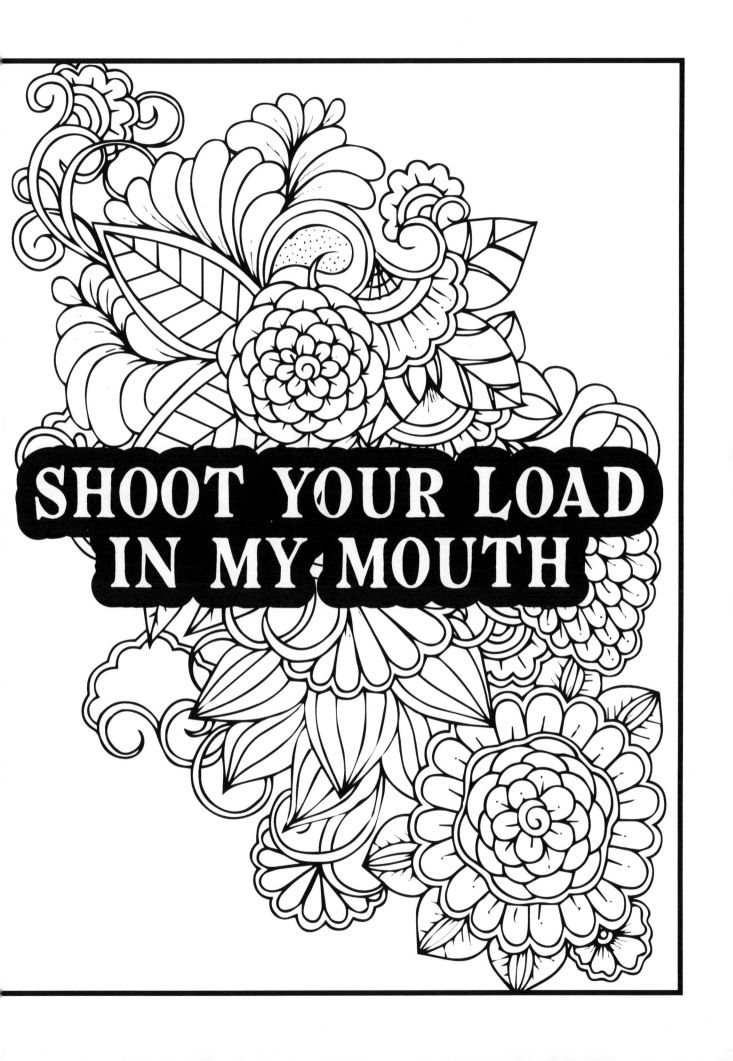

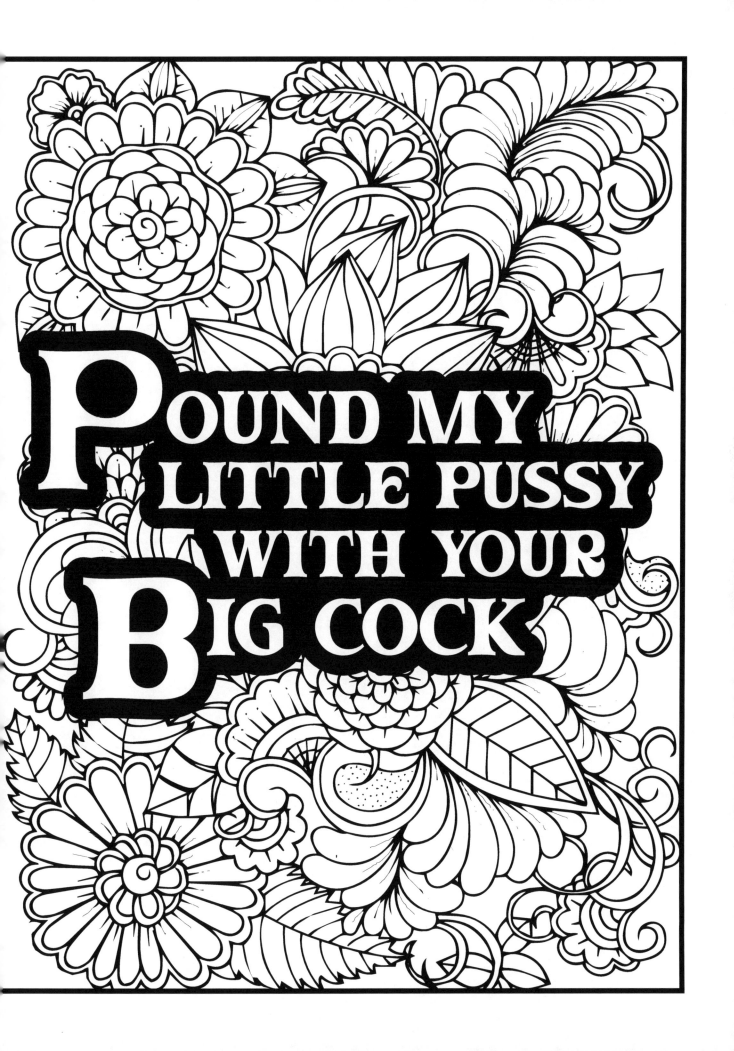

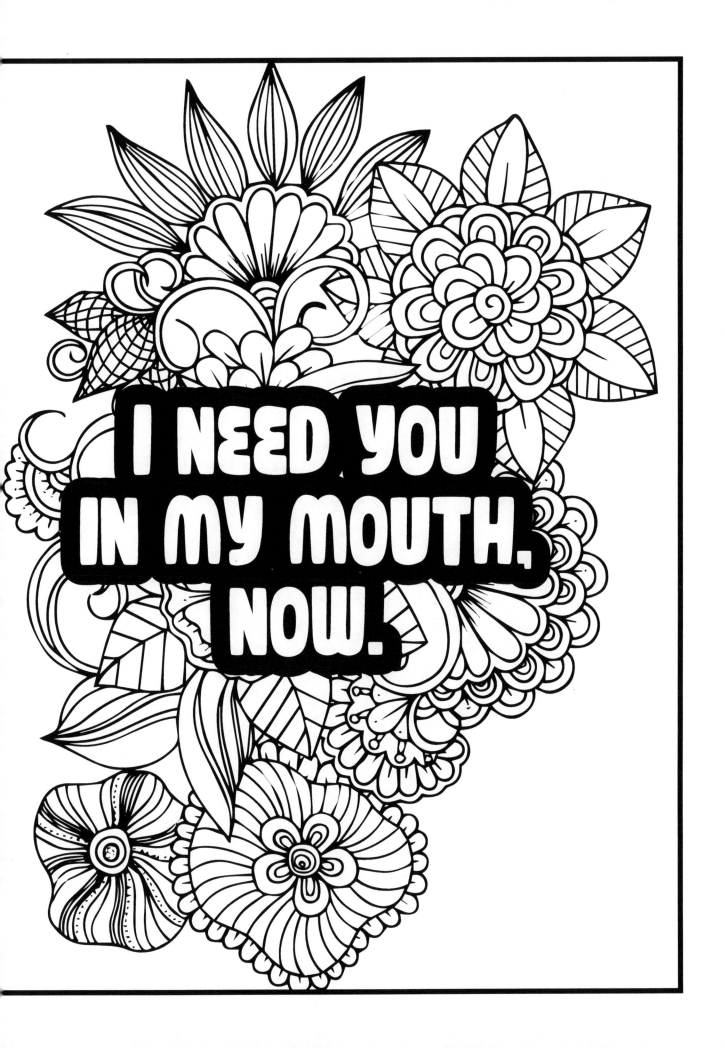

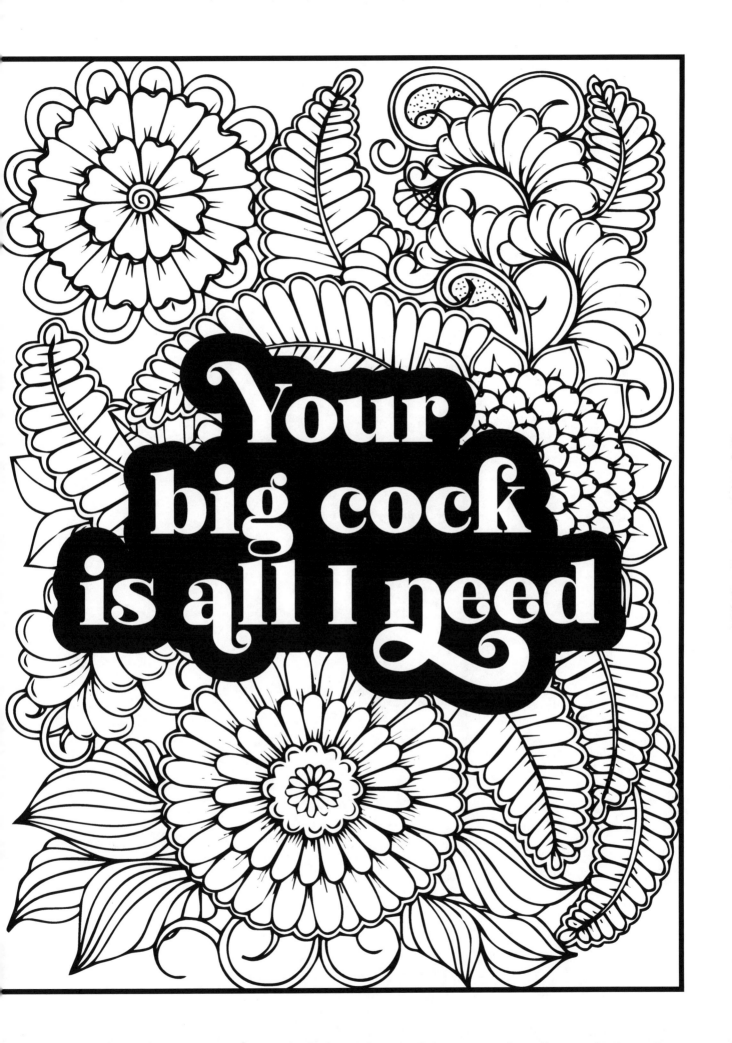

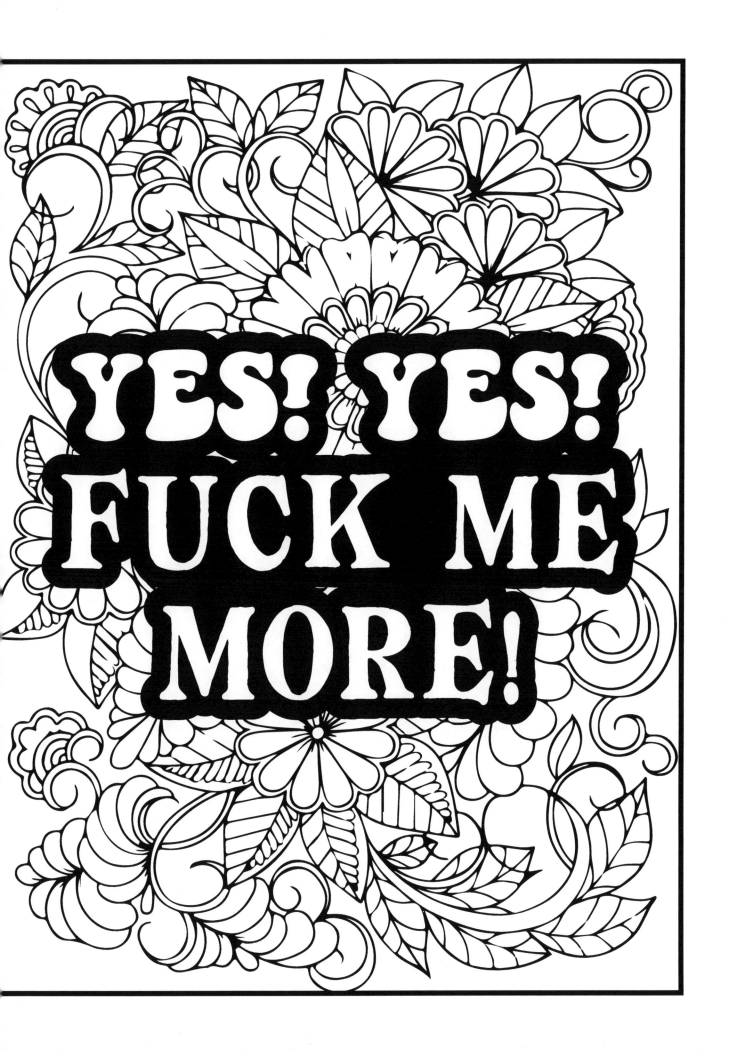

Made in the USA
Monee, IL
02 December 2024

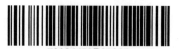

72034450R00037